Simple Explanation of Healthy Nutrition

Hey there, folks!

Welcome to, Simple Explanation of Healthy Nutrition

In a world that's all about fast lifestyles, stress, and unhealthy temptations, it's more important than ever to be mindful of what we eat. We all know that eating healthy is the key to a lively and happy life. But let's be real, sometimes it feels like such a complex and overwhelming topic.

That's why I wrote "Simple Explanation of Healthy Nutrition" - to help you decode the secrets of a balanced and nutrient-rich diet. This book was written with the goal of giving you the knowledge and tools to improve your eating habits and make long-term changes in your life.

And here's the best part: This book ain't your boring nutrition textbook. Nope! We decided to make it entertaining and easy to understand. Each page will take you on an exciting conversation with a virtual nutrition advisor who's here to answer all your questions and give you practical advice.

Whether you're already a nutrition whiz or a newbie in this field, this book is for everyone. From the basics of macros and micros to picking and preparing healthy foods, and even tips for everyday life and sustainable eating habits - we've got everything you need to kickstart or continue your journey to a healthier life.

Now, let me make it clear: this book isn't about strict rules or bans. It's about equipping you with the knowledge and tools to make conscious choices and adapt your eating habits to fit your unique lifestyle. It's all about showing you the joy and possibilities of healthy eating, so you not only feel healthier but also eat with enthusiasm and pleasure.

I hope you see this book as your trusty companion on your path to healthy eating. Use it as your guide, your source of inspiration, and your go-to for answers to all your questions. And most importantly, enjoy it! Because healthy nutrition shouldn't be a drag, but a source of well-being and pure joy.

I wish you loads of fun reading "Healthy Nutrition Made Easy" and hope it inspires you on a lifelong journey to a healthy and fulfilling way of living.

With warm regards,

Kevin van Olafson

Chapter 1: The Importance of Healthy Eating

- Why healthy eating matters
- Effects of poor nutrition on health

Chapter 2: Nutrition Basics

- Macronutrients (carbohydrates, proteins, fats)
- Micronutrients (vitamins, minerals)

Chapter 3: The Role of Fruits and Vegetables

- Why eat fruits and vegetables?
- Tips for selection and preparation

Chapter 4: Whole Grains as a Healthy Choice

- Benefits of whole grain products
- Tips for shopping and usage

Chapter 5: Proteins and Their Sources

- Key sources of protein (meat, fish, legumes)
- Meeting your protein needs

Chapter 6: Healthy Fats and Oils

- Differences between saturated and unsaturated fats
- Healthy fat sources in your diet

Chapter 7: Dairy Products and Alternatives

- Dairy products and their nutrients
- Plant-based alternatives for vegans

Chapter 8: The Importance of Fiber

- Why fiber is important
- Getting to know fiber-rich foods

Chapter 9: Sugar and Sweet Alternatives

- The impact of sugar on health
- Tips for reducing sugar consumption

Chapter 10: Salt and Its Effects

- The role of salt in your diet

<u>*Why healthy eating is crucial:*</u>

Healthy eating is super important for our health and well-being. It plays a big role in preventing diseases, maintaining a healthy weight, and promoting optimal physical and mental performance. But why exactly is healthy eating so important?

First and foremost, a healthy diet provides the necessary nutrients our bodies need to function at their best. Vitamins, minerals, proteins, carbohydrates, and fats are essential for supporting numerous bodily functions. Vitamins and minerals strengthen our immune system, promote cell renewal, and support metabolism. Proteins are the building blocks for muscles, tissues, and enzymes. Carbohydrates are our main source of energy, while fats store important energy and aid in the absorption of fat-soluble vitamins.

In addition, a healthy diet has a positive impact on our weight. A balanced diet with an appropriate calorie intake, combined with physical activity, helps us achieve and maintain a healthy weight. Being overweight or obese is associated with increased risks of various health issues such as heart disease, diabetes, certain types of cancer, and joint problems. By adopting a balanced diet, we can reduce the risk of these diseases and improve our overall health.

Healthy eating also influences our mental performance. Studies have shown that a diet rich in fruits, vegetables, whole grains, healthy fats, and lean protein has positive effects on brain function. These foods provide nutrients that can enhance concentration, memory, and mood. At the same time, they help reduce the risk of neurodegenerative diseases such as Alzheimer's and dementia.

Apart from the individual benefits, healthy eating has broader societal significance. By choosing a healthy diet, we contribute to environmental protection. A plant-rich diet reduces resource consumption, greenhouse gas emissions, and the use of pesticides compared to conventional meat production. Sustainable eating protects our environment and ensures resources for future generations.

A healthy diet can also foster social cohesion. Shared meals offer the opportunity to spend time with family and friends and promote cultural exchange. By practicing mindful food consumption and supporting local producers, we can also strengthen the regional economy.

Overall, healthy eating is a fundamental pillar for a healthy and fulfilling life. It provides our bodies with essential nutrients, supports a healthy weight, enhances mental performance, and contributes to sustainability and social bonding. By making conscious decisions about our diet, we can make the most out of ourselves and contribute to a healthier, happier life.

Impact of Poor Nutrition on Health:

Poor nutrition can have various effects on our health and lead to a range of issues. A diet rich in sugary drinks, fatty snacks, processed foods, and lacking in fruits, vegetables, and whole grains can result in weight gain and eventually obesity. This type of diet often provides many empty calories but few nutrients, causing us to eat more to meet our essential nutrient needs. The excessive calorie intake combined with a lack of physical activity leads to excess energy being stored as fat, resulting in weight gain and ultimately obesity.

Obesity is a serious health problem associated with a variety of diseases and complications. People with obesity have an increased risk of heart disease, strokes, type 2 diabetes, certain types of cancer, high blood pressure, lipid disorders, and joint problems. Additionally, obesity can lead to mental distress such as depression and low self-esteem.

Poor nutrition can also result in an imbalance of nutrients in our bodies. When our diet focuses on processed foods high in sugar and fat, we may not get enough fiber, vitamins, minerals, and antioxidants that are essential for optimal health. This can lead to deficiencies such as iron deficiency, vitamin D deficiency, calcium deficiency, and a lack of essential omega-3 fatty acids.

Unhealthy eating can also increase the risk of cardiovascular diseases. The high content of saturated fats, trans fats, and cholesterol in fatty and processed foods can contribute to the formation of plaque in the arteries, narrowing the blood vessels and increasing the risk of heart attacks and strokes. Moreover, excessive salt intake and an unhealthy diet can lead to high blood pressure, which further increases the risk of cardiovascular diseases.

Another issue of poor nutrition is the increased likelihood of metabolic disorders like type 2 diabetes. A diet high in refined carbohydrates, sugar, and saturated fats can lead to insulin resistance, where cells no longer respond properly to insulin. This results in elevated blood sugar levels and ultimately the development of type 2 diabetes. This condition can lead to severe complications such as kidney disease, eye problems, nerve damage, and cardiovascular diseases.

Lastly, poor nutrition can also impact our mental health. Studies have shown that a diet high in sugar and fat may be associated with an increased risk of depression and anxiety. On the other hand, a balanced diet with sufficient intake of omega-3 fatty acids, antioxidants, and B-vitamins can improve mood and reduce the risk of mental disorders.

Overall, poor nutrition is linked to many negative effects on our health. It can lead to weight gain, obesity, cardiovascular diseases, metabolic disorders, and mental health problems. A balanced diet with adequate nutrient intake from fresh, unprocessed foods is crucial for maintaining health and reducing the risk of diseases.

Chapter 2: Basics of Nutrition

Macronutrients (Carbohydrates, Proteins, Fats):

Macronutrients are the key players in our diet, providing us with the energy and building blocks our body needs to function optimally. The three main macronutrients are carbohydrates, proteins, and fats. Each of them has different functions and impacts on our body. Here's a detailed and interesting explanation of macronutrients:

Carbohydrates:

Carbs are the primary source of energy for our body. They consist of sugar molecules that are broken down into glucose in the digestive system. Glucose is then used by our cells to produce energy. Carbohydrates come in various forms, including simple carbs (like sugar) and complex carbs (like starch and fiber). Complex carbohydrates found in whole grains, legumes, and vegetables are digested more slowly, providing a sustained energy supply. Fiber, a type of carbohydrate, promotes gut health, regulates blood sugar levels, and contributes to satiety. Consuming a balanced amount of carbohydrates is important to have enough energy for physical activities and metabolic processes.

Proteins:

Proteins are essential building blocks for our body. They consist of amino acids, some of which our body cannot produce on its own and therefore must be obtained through food. Proteins have many important functions: they are responsible for tissue growth and repair, support muscle, enzyme, and hormone production, enhance immune function, and help maintain acid-base balance.

Proteins are found in animal sources like meat, fish, eggs, and dairy products, as well as plant sources like legumes, nuts, seeds, and grains. A balanced diet should include an adequate amount of proteins to meet the body's needs. It's important to consider both the quantity and quality of proteins, as animal proteins contain all essential amino acids, while plant proteins should be consumed in combination to cover all amino acids.

Fats:

Fats are an important source of energy for our body and serve various functions. They aid in the absorption of fat-soluble vitamins (like vitamin A, D, E, and K), insulate our body and protect our organs, promote hormone production, and serve as an energy reserve.

There are different types of fats, including saturated fats, unsaturated fats, and trans fats. Saturated fats, mainly found in animal products and some plant oils, should be consumed in moderation as they are associated with an increased risk of cardiovascular diseases. Unsaturated fats found in foods like nuts, seeds, avocados, and plant oils, on the other hand, are beneficial to health and should be included in the diet.

It's important to note that fats have a higher energy density than carbohydrates and proteins. Therefore, their intake should be in appropriate amounts to maintain a healthy body weight. Striking a balance between saturated and unsaturated fats and avoiding trans fats is crucial.

A balanced diet should include all three macronutrients in appropriate amounts to provide the body with energy and support various bodily functions. It's important to focus on the quality of food and choose a variety of healthy sources for carbohydrates, proteins, and fats to promote optimal health and well-being.

Micronutrients (Vitamins, Minerals):

While micronutrients are required in small quantities, they play a crucial role in our health. Vitamins and minerals are the two main categories of micronutrients and fulfill a variety of functions in the body. Here's a detailed explanation of the importance of vitamins and minerals for our health:

Vitamins:

Vitamins are organic compounds essential for maintaining smooth operation of numerous metabolic processes and bodily functions. There are two main categories of vitamins: fat-soluble vitamins (vitamin A, D, E, and K) and water-soluble vitamins (vitamin C and B-vitamins).
Fat-soluble vitamins dissolve in fat and can be stored in the body. They are essential for the health of the skin, bones, eyes, immune system, and reproductive system. Vitamin A is important for vision and maintaining healthy skin. It also plays a role in cell development and reproduction. Vitamin D is essential for the absorption of calcium and phosphorus, thus crucial for strong bones and teeth. Vitamin E is a potent antioxidant that protects cells from damage caused by free radicals. Vitamin K is important for blood clotting and contributes to bone health.

Water-soluble vitamins are not stored in the body and need to be regularly consumed through food. They are involved in numerous metabolic processes and play a role in energy production, cell growth, nervous system function, and immune support. Vitamin C is a strong antioxidant that strengthens the immune function and contributes to collagen formation. The B-vitamins, including B1 (thiamine), B2 (riboflavin), B6 (pyridoxine), B12 (cobalamin), and folic acid, are important for energy metabolism, formation of red blood cells, and supporting the nervous system.

Minerals:

Minerals are inorganic substances that are essential for many bodily functions and biochemical processes. They are divided into two main categories: major minerals (such as calcium, magnesium, potassium, sodium, and phosphorus) and trace minerals (such as iron, zinc, copper, iodine, and selenium).
Major minerals are required in larger amounts and play a crucial role in maintaining healthy bone and muscle tissue, regulating fluid balance, controlling blood pressure, and supporting the nervous system. Calcium is essential for strong bones and teeth. It is also involved in cell signaling and muscle contraction. Magnesium is involved in over 300 enzymatic reactions in the body and supports energy metabolism, muscle and nerve function, and bone health.

Trace minerals are needed in small amounts but are still crucial for our health. They play a role in enzyme and hormone production, immune support, energy production, and cell function. Iron is responsible for oxygen transport in the body and plays an important role in the formation of red blood cells. Zinc is involved in numerous enzymatic reactions and contributes to wound healing and immune system strengthening. Copper is important for connective tissue formation and iron utilization. Iodine is essential for thyroid function and production of thyroid hormones.

Selenium is an antioxidant that protects cells from damage caused by free radicals and supports the immune system.

Vitamins and minerals are essential for optimal health and should be obtained through a balanced diet or supplementation if needed. A variety of fresh fruits, vegetables, whole grains, lean meats, fish, nuts, and seeds can ensure that the body receives the necessary micronutrients. It's important to focus on a balanced and varied diet to ensure that all vitamins and minerals are adequately present and able to fulfill their respective functions in the body.

Chapter 3: The Role of Fruits and Vegetables

Why Eat Fruits and Veggies?

Fruits and veggies are like super-packed nutrient bombs that are really good for your health. They have lots of vitamins, minerals, fiber, and stuff called antioxidants that are super important. Vitamins like C, A, and the B ones are all in there. Vitamin C helps your immune system, heals wounds, and helps make collagen for your skin. Vitamin A is awesome for your eyes and skin. And the B vitamins are all about energy, blood cells, and keeping your nerves in check.

And get this—fruits and veggies are also packed with minerals like potassium, magnesium, and iron. Potassium keeps your blood pressure in check, magnesium does like 300 cool things in your body, and iron is all about making red blood cells and delivering oxygen.

Fiber is another thing fruits and veggies have. It's really good for your digestion and helps regulate blood sugar, keeps your heart healthy, and helps with weight management. Basically, eating fiber-rich foods like fruits and veggies can make you feel full and keep those cravings in check.

But wait, there's more! Fruits and veggies have a ton of antioxidants. These are like superheroes that protect your cells from damage caused by things like pollution, stress, and junky food. Too many free radicals can mess things up and make you more likely to get sick or age faster. But by eating fruits and veggies with antioxidants like vitamins C and E, and beta-carotene, you can fight off those bad guys and stay healthy.

Oh, and remember to mix it up! Different fruits and veggies have different nutrients. Green leafy stuff like spinach and kale have iron and vitamin K, while orange goodies like carrots and sweet potatoes have beta-carotene, which your body turns into vitamin A. So, eating a variety of fruits and veggies is like giving your body a buffet of awesome nutrients.

And get this—eating fruits and veggies can lower your risk of getting sick. Lots of studies have shown that people who eat fruits and veggies regularly have a lower risk of heart disease, certain cancers, stroke, and type 2 diabetes. All those vitamins, fiber, and antioxidants can help lower cholesterol, regulate blood pressure, reduce inflammation, and keep your blood sugar in check.

So, make sure to choose fresh, high-quality fruits and veggies. Don't store them for too long or cook them to death, though, 'cause that can zap the nutrients. Try eating them raw or lightly cooked to get the most out of their good stuff.

To sum it up, fruits and veggies are essential for a healthy diet. They're full of important nutrients, fiber, and antioxidants that keep you in tip-top shape. By eating them regularly, you'll boost your immune system, reduce the risk of diseases, keep your digestion happy, and maintain a healthy weight. So, don't forget to make fruits and veggies a part of your balanced diet.

Tips for Picking and Prepping:

This chapter not only tells you how awesome fruits and veggies are but also gives you some handy tips on how to pick and prep them. Check it out:

1. Picking Fruits and Veggies:

Choose fresh fruits and veggies that are ripe, firm, and free from yucky spots or damage. Try to go for different varieties and colors to get a wide range of nutrients. And go for seasonal produce whenever possible—they're usually fresher and tastier.

2. Go Organic:

If you can, opt for organic fruits and veggies. They're grown without synthetic pesticides and herbicides, so they might be a healthier choice. But remember, conventionally grown ones still have plenty of health benefits too.

3. Storing:

Store your fruits and veggies right to keep them fresh and nutritious for longer. Some, like apples, bananas, and tomatoes, can be kept at room temperature, while others like berries, lettuce, and herbs should go in the fridge. Don't store them for too long, though, 'cause that can make them lose nutrients.

4. Cooking Methods:

There are lots of ways to cook fruits and veggies while keeping their nutrients intact and making them taste great. You can eat them raw as a snack or in salads for a crunchy and fresh addition. They can also be steamed, sautéed, grilled, or used in soups and stews. But keep in mind that longer cooking times can reduce the water-soluble vitamins, so gentler cooking methods are better.

5. Preserve Texture:

When cooking fruits and veggies, it's important to preserve their texture for a more enjoyable eating experience. Avoid overcooking, which can turn them mushy. Instead, try blanching or steaming them briefly to maintain their crispness and color. You can also use different cutting techniques like dicing, julienning, or spiralizing to add variety and visual appeal to your plate.

6. Get Creative:

Don't be afraid to experiment and get creative with cooking fruits and veggies. You can use them in smoothies, juices, soups, casseroles, pasta dishes, wraps, and so much more. Try out new recipes and explore different flavors and combinations.

7. Adding to Other Dishes:

Boost your fruit and veggie intake by adding them to other dishes. For example, you can chop veggies and add them to omelets, salads, sandwiches, or wraps. Use fruits as toppings for yogurt, oats, or pancakes. You can also sneak veggies into soups, stews, sauces, or casseroles to increase the nutritional value of your meals.

By following these tips for selecting and preparing fruits and veggies, you'll ensure you get the full health benefits of these essential foods. Enjoy the variety of flavors, textures, and colors they offer and make them a staple of your balanced diet.

<u>Chapter 4: Whole Grain Products as a Healthy Choice</u>

<u>Benefits of Whole Grain Products:</u>

The chapter "Whole Grain Products as a Healthy Choice" talks about why whole grain products are a good option for our health and the many advantages they offer. Whole grain products are foods that use the whole grain, including the inner part, germ, and bran. On the other hand, refined grain products are made by removing the outer layer, bran, and germ, which results in the loss of important nutrients.

One big benefit of whole grain products is that they are rich in fiber. Fiber is a type of carbohydrate that our body can't fully digest. You can find fiber in whole grain products like whole wheat bread, whole wheat pasta, brown rice, oats, and quinoa. Fiber is great for promoting good digestion by improving bowel movements and regulating stool consistency. It can prevent constipation and make sure our bowel movements happen regularly and easily.

Fiber also helps control blood sugar levels. Compared to refined grain products, whole grain products are digested and absorbed more slowly. This means our blood sugar levels rise more slowly after a meal, which can be helpful for people with diabetes or those who want to prevent it. Having stable blood sugar levels can also prevent cravings and help us feel full for a longer time.

Another advantage of whole grain products is their high content of essential vitamins and minerals. Whole grain products contain various nutrients such as B vitamins (like thiamin, riboflavin, niacin, B6, and folic acid), vitamin E, iron, magnesium, zinc, and selenium. These nutrients are important for our overall health and play a role in different functions in our body.

B vitamins in whole grain products are crucial for energy metabolism and supporting our nervous system. Vitamin E is an antioxidant that protects our cells from damage caused by free radicals. Iron is important for forming red blood cells and transporting oxygen in our body. Magnesium supports muscle and nerve function and helps maintain healthy bones. Zinc plays a role in supporting our immune system and wound healing. Selenium is a trace element with antioxidant properties that contributes to our cellular health.

Eating whole grain products can also reduce the risk of chronic diseases. Many studies have shown that people who regularly consume whole grain products have a lower risk of heart disease, strokes, certain types of cancer (like colon cancer), and type 2 diabetes. This is partly because of the health-promoting properties of fiber, vitamins, minerals, and other beneficial compounds found in whole grain products.

Moreover, whole grain products have a high satiety effect. This means they keep us feeling full for a longer time and can reduce cravings. This can be especially helpful for people who want to lose weight or maintain their weight. By including whole grain products in our diet, we can feel energized and satisfied for longer periods without constantly reaching for snacks.

To fully enjoy the benefits of whole grain products, it's important to incorporate them into our meals. Instead of choosing refined grain products like white bread, white pasta, and white rice, go for whole grain alternatives like whole wheat bread, whole wheat pasta, and brown rice. Try different whole grain products like quinoa, bulgur, millet, and oats to add variety and flavor to your meals.

There are many ways to prepare and enjoy whole grain products. They can be served as side dishes, such as whole wheat pasta with tomato sauce or brown rice with steamed vegetables and chicken. They can also be added to salads by including ingredients like oats or quinoa in green leafy salads. And of course, you can enhance your breakfast by enjoying oatmeal or whole grain cereal with yogurt and fresh fruit.

By making whole grain products a regular part of your diet, you can experience the numerous health benefits they offer. From better digestion and stable blood sugar control to reducing the risk of chronic diseases, whole grain products contribute to a balanced diet and overall good health. Enjoy the variety of whole grain options and experiment with new recipes to make your meals diverse and delicious.

Tips for Shopping and Usage:

Whole grain products are an awesome choice to support a healthy diet and offer a bunch of benefits for our health. Unlike refined grain products, which have the nutrient-rich germ and bran layers removed, whole grain products contain all parts of the grain - the germ, bran, and endosperm. That's why they're packed with fiber, vitamins, minerals, and other essential nutrients our bodies need to function optimally.

Fiber is a key component of whole grain products. It helps promote a healthy digestion by regulating stool consistency and preventing constipation. Fiber also helps stabilize blood sugar levels by slowing down the absorption of glucose. This is particularly beneficial for people with diabetes or those who want to manage their blood sugar levels. Additionally, fiber contributes to lowering cholesterol levels and reducing the risk of heart disease.

Whole grain products are also a rich source of various vitamins and minerals that are essential for optimal health. They contain a variety of B vitamins like thiamin, riboflavin, niacin, and folic acid, which play important roles in energy metabolism, nervous system function, and red blood cell formation. Furthermore, whole grain products provide minerals like magnesium, iron, zinc, and selenium, which are crucial for supporting the immune system, bone health, and numerous other bodily functions.

Regular consumption of whole grain products can also offer long-term health benefits. Studies have shown that people who have a diet high in whole grain products have a lower risk of chronic diseases. These include heart disease, strokes, type 2 diabetes, and certain types of cancer like colon cancer. This is partially due to the antioxidants, phytochemicals, and other bioactive compounds present in whole grain products, which have anti-inflammatory properties and can protect our cells from damage.

To make the most of the benefits of whole grain products, it's important to integrate various options into your diet. There's a wide variety of whole grain products to choose from, including whole grain bread, whole wheat pasta, brown rice, oats, quinoa, and whole grain cereals. Get creative and try out new recipes to discover the diversity of whole grain products. For example, you can prepare a colorful salad with quinoa, enjoy whole wheat pasta with a tasty vegetable sauce, or start your day with a bowl of oatmeal topped with fresh fruit.

When shopping for whole grain products, pay attention to the labels and look for products labeled as "whole grain" or "100% whole grain." This ensures that you're actually getting products made from whole grain and reaping all the health benefits. When storing whole grain products at home, it's important to keep them in airtight containers in a cool, dry, and dark place to maintain their freshness and quality.

Incorporating whole grain products into your diet is an easy and delicious way to improve your health while obtaining a variety of nutrients. Start slowly and take small steps to introduce more whole grain products into your meals. For example, you can replace refined grain products with whole grain alternatives, choose whole grain bread over white bread, or use oats as a base for your breakfast. Over time, you'll notice improvements in your well-being and enjoy the benefits of a wholesome diet rich in whole grain products.

<u>Chapter 5: Proteins and Their Sources</u>

<u>*Important Protein Sources (Meat, Fish, Legumes)*</u>*:*

Proteins are essential nutrients that play a vital role in building and maintaining tissues and organs in our bodies. They are the building blocks of cells, muscles, bones, skin, hair, and nails. In addition to their structural function, proteins also support metabolism, the immune system, and the production of enzymes and hormones. It is therefore crucial to include sufficient protein in our diet to ensure optimal health and functioning of our bodies.

There are various sources of proteins, and a balanced diet should include a variety of protein sources. Meat and poultry are traditional protein sources that are rich in essential amino acids. They provide high-quality animal protein and are particularly rich in B vitamins, iron, zinc, and other important nutrients. Red meat such as beef, lamb, and pork is a good source of iron, while poultry such as chicken and turkey have less fat and cholesterol. However, it is important to choose lean meats and consider cooking methods to control the fat content.

Fish and seafood are also excellent protein sources. They contain high-quality animal protein as well as omega-3 fatty acids, which have anti-inflammatory properties and are beneficial for heart health. Fatty fish species like salmon, mackerel, tuna, and sardines are particularly rich in omega-3 fatty acids. Additionally, fish and seafood are rich in minerals such as iodine, selenium, and zinc. Regular consumption of fish in the diet can help reduce the risk of heart disease, stroke, and certain types of cancer.

Legumes such as beans, lentils, chickpeas, and peas are excellent plant-based protein sources. They not only provide protein but also contain fiber, complex carbohydrates, and a variety of vitamins and minerals. Legumes are also rich in phytochemicals, which have strong antioxidant properties and can act as anti-inflammatory agents. They are an excellent choice for vegetarians and vegans who want to meet their protein needs from plant sources. Legumes can be used in various dishes such as stews, salads, curries, and patties, offering a diverse and tasty way to enrich the diet.

It is important to note that in a balanced diet, diversity of protein sources is crucial. In addition to meat, fish, and legumes, there are also other sources such as dairy products, eggs, nuts, and seeds. Each protein source offers different nutrients and health benefits. Therefore, it is advisable to include various protein sources in your meals to obtain a complete range of essential amino acids and other nutrients.

Choosing high-quality protein sources is important to achieve the best results for your health. Make sure to choose lean meats, remove the skin from poultry, and prefer fatty fish varieties. When it comes to plant-based protein sources, it is important to combine different varieties to ensure a complete amino acid composition. If you follow a vegetarian or vegan diet, you can also incorporate plant-based substitutes like tofu, tempeh, and seitan into your diet.

Overall, it is important to recognize the importance of proteins in our diet and ensure that we obtain sufficient amounts from various sources. By choosing a variety of protein sources, we can ensure that we receive all the necessary amino acids and nutrients required for optimal health and functioning of our bodies.

Proteins are made up of amino acids, which serve as building blocks to form tissues and organs in our body. There are a total of 20 amino acids, nine of which are considered essential as our bodies cannot produce them on their own and we need to consume them through food. Adequate intake of high-quality proteins ensures that our body receives all the essential amino acids it needs.

In addition to meat, fish, and legumes, there are other protein sources that can be considered in a healthy diet. Dairy products such as milk, yogurt, and cheese are rich in high-quality animal protein and also contain important nutrients such as calcium and vitamin D. Eggs are also an excellent source of protein and provide a wide range of vitamins and minerals.

If you are interested in plant-based protein sources, you can turn to nuts and seeds. Almonds, walnuts, cashews, chia seeds, and flaxseeds are just a few examples of protein-rich plant-based foods. These not only provide protein but also healthy fats, fiber, and a variety of vitamins and minerals.

Another aspect to consider when selecting protein sources is the quality of the protein. Biological value indicates how well the body can utilize the protein from a particular source. Animal proteins generally have a higher biological value than plant proteins as they have a complete amino acid composition. For plant-based protein sources, it is important to combine different varieties to achieve a balanced amino acid composition.

The preparation of protein-rich foods can also affect their nutrient composition. Grilling, frying, or cooking meat can lead to changes in protein structure. Some cooking methods may increase fat content, while others preserve important nutrients. Therefore, it is advisable to choose healthier cooking methods such as steaming, roasting, or grilling instead of opting for fried or heavily processed options.

Overall, the selection of protein-rich foods is of great importance for a balanced diet and optimal health. You should aim to include a variety of protein sources in your meals to ensure that you receive all essential amino acids and nutrients. A balanced diet with high-quality proteins can help build muscle mass, support metabolism, strengthen the immune system, and promote a general sense of satiety.

How to Meet Your Protein Needs:

Proteins are super important nutrients that play a big role in our bodies. They're like the building blocks for our tissues, muscles, organs, and enzymes, and they're involved in a bunch of biological processes. So, to make sure we're meeting our protein needs and keeping our bodies in tip-top shape, it's important to know how to choose the right protein sources and incorporate them into our diet.

The amount of protein we need can vary from person to person and depends on things like age, gender, physical activity, and individual needs. As a general recommendation, adults should aim for about 0.8 grams of protein per kilogram of body weight per day. However, if you're active, an athlete, or looking to build muscle, you might need more protein.

To meet your protein needs, your diet should include a variety of protein-rich foods. Meat and poultry are traditional protein sources. Lean meats like chicken, turkey, beef, and pork contain high-quality animal protein and provide important nutrients like iron and B-vitamins. Fish and seafood are also excellent sources of protein. Fatty fish like salmon, mackerel, and tuna not only deliver high-quality protein but also healthy omega-3 fatty acids, which have anti-inflammatory properties and promote heart health.

For folks who don't consume animal products, legumes such as beans, lentils, chickpeas, and peas are important protein sources. They're also rich in fiber and packed with various vitamins and minerals. Legumes can be used in soups, stews, salads, or as a main ingredient in vegetarian dishes. They're a great alternative to meat and can support a healthy, protein-rich diet.

Dairy products like milk, yogurt, and cheese are also important protein sources, especially for those who don't consume animal products. They provide high-quality animal protein as well as calcium and vitamin D, which are important for strong bones and teeth. Eggs are a versatile protein source and also provide essential vitamins and minerals like Vitamin B12 and choline.

In addition to the main sources mentioned, there are also plant-based protein sources like tofu, tempeh, quinoa, nuts, seeds, and whole grains. These not only provide protein but also healthy fats, fiber, and other nutrients. Plant-based proteins are also suitable for vegetarians and vegans and can be a great option for meeting protein needs.

It's important to vary your protein sources in meals to ensure a balanced amino acid composition. By combining different protein sources, you can make sure you're getting all the essential amino acids your body needs. For example, you can combine legumes with whole grains to create a complete protein source. Combining plant-based and animal protein sources can also be a good option for achieving a balanced diet.

There are different ways to prepare protein-rich foods. Meats and fish can be grilled, fried, steamed, or baked. When cooking legumes, make sure to cook them adequately to improve their digestibility. Plant-based protein sources like tofu and tempeh can be fried, marinated, or incorporated into various dishes. It's also important to combine protein sources with a variety of vegetables, whole grains, and healthy fats to create a balanced meal.

Overall, it's important to consider your individual protein needs and promote a diverse diet to ensure adequate protein intake. A balanced mix of animal and plant-based protein sources, combined with a variety of healthy ingredients, can help promote health and well-being and provide your body with the necessary building blocks to function properly.

Chapter 6: Healthy Fats and Oils

Differences between Saturated and Unsaturated Fatty Acids:

Healthy fats and oils play a crucial role in our diet and are important for our health. They serve not only as a significant source of energy but also fulfill various other functions in our bodies. Specifically, they are essential for the absorption of fat-soluble vitamins such as vitamins A, D, E, and K. Additionally, fats and oils are involved in the formation of cell membranes and serve as precursors for hormone production. However, to maximize the benefits of fats and minimize the risks associated with certain fatty acids, it is important to understand the difference between saturated and unsaturated fatty acids.

Saturated fatty acids are found in animal products such as meat, butter, cheese, and cream. They are also present in some plant sources like coconut oil and palm oil. Saturated fatty acids have been criticized in the past due to their potential negative impact on heart health. Excessive consumption of saturated fats can raise cholesterol levels and increase the risk of cardiovascular diseases. Therefore, it is recommended to limit the intake of saturated fatty acids and replace them with healthier options.

On the other hand, unsaturated fatty acids are known as healthy fats and play a crucial role in our diet. They are primarily found in plant oils such as olive oil, canola oil, sunflower oil, and avocado oil. They are also present in nuts, seeds, and certain types of fish. Unsaturated fatty acids are liquid at room temperature and have a favorable effect on our cardiovascular health. They can help lower cholesterol levels, reduce inflammation in the body, and decrease the risk of cardiovascular diseases.

There are two types of unsaturated fatty acids: monounsaturated fatty acids and polyunsaturated fatty acids. Monounsaturated fatty acids are mainly found in olive oil, avocado, almonds, and cashews. They are characterized by their anti-inflammatory properties and can contribute to maintaining a healthy heart. Polyunsaturated fatty acids are rich in omega-3 and omega-6 fatty acids and are found in fatty fish like salmon, mackerel, and sardines, as well as in flaxseeds, chia seeds, and walnuts. Omega-3 fatty acids are known for their positive effects on brain function, heart health, and reducing inflammation in the body. Omega-6 fatty acids are also important but should be consumed in the proper ratio to omega-3 fatty acids to maintain an optimal balance.

When choosing healthy fats and oils, it is important to pay attention to their quality. High-quality cold-pressed oils that have been produced gently and retain their natural color and flavors are the best choice. Refined oils, on the other hand, undergo a series of processing steps and may be less healthy. It is also important to avoid trans fats as they can increase the risk of heart diseases. Trans fats are found in many processed foods such as baked goods, snacks, and fried foods.

To maximize the benefits of healthy fats in your diet, you can replace saturated fats with unsaturated fats. For example, use olive oil instead of butter when cooking and dressing. Avocado is a great option to incorporate healthy fats into salads, sandwiches, or smoothies. Consuming fatty fish like salmon or mackerel two to three times a week is a good way to obtain omega-3 fatty acids. Nuts and seeds can be used as snacks or as toppings for cereals and yogurt, providing a rich source of unsaturated fats.

Overall, it is important to find a balanced ratio between saturated and unsaturated fatty acids and consider the quality of fats and oils used. By making conscious choices and using healthy fats, you can support your health and enhance the taste and diversity of your meals. Remember that while fats play an important role in our diet, they are also high in calories. Therefore, be mindful of consuming them in moderation and combine them with an overall balanced diet and a healthy lifestyle.

Healthy Fat Sources in Your Diet:

Healthy fats and oils are an essential part of a balanced diet and play a crucial role in our health. Fat is an important source of energy for our bodies and helps with the absorption of fat-soluble vitamins. Additionally, they are important for hormone production and contribute to the formation of cell membranes. However, there are differences between different types of fats, and it is important to choose the right sources of healthy fats in our diet.

A good source of healthy fats is plant oils. Olive oil, canola oil, avocado oil, and coconut oil are examples of healthy options. These oils mainly contain unsaturated fatty acids, especially monounsaturated fatty acids. These fats are beneficial for heart health as they can help lower cholesterol levels and reduce inflammation in the body. They are also rich in antioxidants, which can help prevent cell damage.

In addition to plant oils, nuts and seeds are also good sources of healthy fats. Almonds, walnuts, cashews, chia seeds, flaxseeds, and sunflower seeds are rich in unsaturated fatty acids and offer a variety of health benefits. They can be eaten as snacks, sprinkled on salads, or added to smoothies.

Fatty fish such as salmon, mackerel, tuna, and sardines are also good sources of healthy fats. These fish are rich in omega-3 fatty acids, which have anti-inflammatory properties and are important for heart and brain health. Regular consumption of fatty fish can reduce the risk of heart diseases and improve cognitive function.

It is also important to limit the consumption of saturated fats. Saturated fats are mainly found in animal products such as meat, full-fat dairy products, and butter. High intake of saturated fats can increase the risk of cardiovascular diseases. It is recommended to choose lean meats, remove the skin from poultry, and reduce the consumption of high-fat dairy products.

When preparing meals, it is advisable to choose healthy fat sources. Use plant oils instead of butter or other saturated fats for cooking and frying. Try to avoid fried foods and opt for healthier cooking methods such as steaming, grilling, or baking.

It is important to note that fats still have a high energy density, which means they contain a lot of calories. Excessive fat intake can lead to weight gain. Therefore, be mindful of consuming a moderate amount of fat in your diet and combine it with an overall balanced diet and a healthy lifestyle.

By incorporating healthy fat sources into your diet, you can benefit from the many advantages of healthy fats. They not only support heart and brain health but also contribute to overall health and well-being. Making conscious choices of healthy fat sources and preparing meals correctly can help you achieve a healthy and balanced diet.

Chapter 7: Dairy Products and Alternatives

Dairy Products and Their Goodies:

Dairy products are super versatile and important in our diet. They not only taste great but also give us a bunch of nutrients that are super important for our health. From classic dairy products like milk, yogurt, and cheese to cool plant-based alternatives, there are lots of options to choose from based on what you like and need.

Dairy products are awesome because they're packed with calcium, protein, and vitamins. Calcium is crucial for strong bones and teeth, and dairy products, especially milk, have lots of easily absorbable calcium. It's especially important for kids and teens when their bones are growing. But even as adults, calcium helps prevent brittle bones and stuff like osteoporosis.

Plus, dairy products have loads of protein, which is important for building and repairing tissues, making enzymes and hormones, and keeping our immune system strong. Yogurt and cheese have high-quality proteins that give us all the essential amino acids we need. That's great for vegetarians and vegans looking for alternative protein sources.

Dairy products also give us a bunch of vitamins and minerals that keep us healthy. Vitamin B12, found in milk and cheese, helps make red blood cells and keeps our nervous system working right. Riboflavin (Vitamin B2) helps with lots of important body processes and keeps our skin and eyes healthy. And let's not forget about vitamin D, which helps us absorb and use calcium for strong bones and muscles.

If you're lactose intolerant or just prefer plant-based options for ethical, health, or environmental reasons, there are plenty of plant-based milk alternatives out there. Oat milk, almond milk, soy milk, coconut milk—you've got choices! They're made from plants and don't have lactose. They're a good option for folks with cow's milk allergies or those who choose to skip animal products.

Just remember that plant-based alternatives might not have all the same nutrients as dairy products. Some might have less protein, for example. So, check the labels and look for fortified versions with added calcium, vitamin D, and B12 to make sure you're still getting the good stuff.

When you're picking dairy products or plant-based alternatives, keep an eye on the fat content too. Full-fat dairy products have more saturated fats, while low-fat or fat-free options have less fat. Yogurt with live cultures is a particularly good choice because it has probiotic bacteria that are good for your gut. Cheese is tasty, but enjoy it in moderation because it can be higher in fat, even though it's packed with calcium and protein.

Remember, moderation is key! Dairy products or their alternatives are just part of a balanced diet. Make sure you're eating a variety of foods. If you have any questions or specific dietary needs, talk to a registered dietitian or doctor to get personalized advice.

All in all, dairy products and their alternatives give us lots of options to get the calcium, protein, and other nutrients we need. Make smart choices, watch the fat content, and enjoy the benefits of this food group for a healthy diet.

Plant-based alternatives for vegans:

For people who choose a vegan diet, there are a variety of plant-based and other alternatives to dairy products that allow them to meet their nutritional needs without consuming animal products. These alternatives not only offer a wide range of flavors but also provide important nutrients and can be used in many recipes and dishes.

One of the most popular plant-based milk alternatives is soy milk. It is made from soybeans and offers an excellent source of protein, calcium, and vitamin D. Soy milk has a mild taste and a creamy consistency, making it a great option for use in coffee, tea, smoothies, and baked goods. It is also available in fortified form, meaning it is enriched with additional nutrients like vitamins and minerals to ensure vegans get the necessary nutrients.

Another popular alternative is almond milk. It is made from ground almonds and water, offering a delicious nutty flavor. Almond milk is rich in vitamin E, magnesium, and unsaturated fats. It works well for people with lactose intolerance or milk allergies and can be used in many recipes and beverages. Almond milk is also available in different flavors like vanilla or chocolate to cater to individual preferences.

Oat milk is also a popular choice for vegans. It is made from oats and water and has a mild, slightly sweet taste. Oat milk is rich in fiber, vitamins, and minerals like iron and magnesium. It works well for people with gluten intolerance as it is naturally gluten-free. Oat milk is a versatile alternative that can be used in coffee, tea, cereal, and smoothies. It can also be used for baking and cooking to provide a creamy texture and a slightly sweet taste.

Coconut milk is another option commonly used in vegan cuisine. It is made from the flesh of coconuts and offers a creamy taste with a hint of exotic flavor. Coconut milk contains healthy fats and provides a good source of iron and magnesium. It can be used in soups, curries, desserts, and beverages, adding richness and creaminess to dishes. In addition to coconut milk, there are also coconut yogurts and other coconut-based products that serve as tasty alternatives to conventional dairy products.

In addition to plant-based alternatives, there are other options for vegans as well. Rice milk, for example, is made from rice and has a mild and sweet taste. It is naturally lactose-free and gluten-free but has less protein compared to other milk alternatives. Rice milk works well for people with allergies or intolerances to soy, nuts, or oats.

Another option is nut milk alternatives like cashew milk, hazelnut milk, or macadamia milk. These are made from ground nuts and water, offering a creamy taste and a good source of healthy fats. They are rich in vitamins and minerals and can be used in various recipes and beverages.

Vegans can also turn to other plant sources for dairy alternatives, such as hemp milk. It is made from hemp seeds and has a nutty taste. Hemp milk is rich in omega-3 fatty acids and provides a good source of plant-based protein. It is also a good option for people with allergies or intolerances.

When selecting plant-based or other alternatives, it is important to pay attention to quality and the ingredient list. Some commercial products may contain additives or sweeteners, so it is advisable to look for organic options or prepare your own alternatives at home. This allows you to maintain control over the ingredients and ensure you enjoy high-quality and healthy alternatives to dairy products.

Overall, plant-based and other alternatives to dairy products offer a great way for vegans to meet their nutritional needs while still enjoying a varied and delicious diet. By trying out different options and selecting those that best suit personal taste and individual needs, one can achieve a healthy and balanced plant-based diet.

Chapter 8: The Importance of Fiber

Why Fiber Matters:

Fiber is super important for a healthy diet and keeping our digestion in check. It's a type of carb found in plants that our bodies can't fully break down. Instead, it mostly passes through our digestive system unchanged, but that's actually a good thing.

One of the main things fiber does is keep our gut healthy. It adds bulk to our stool and makes it softer, so we can avoid getting all blocked up and have smooth trips to the bathroom. Fiber also helps our intestines move things along, so we can have regular and easy poops. And when our digestive system is happy, we reduce the risk of problems like colon cancer and painful hemorrhoids.

But that's not all fiber does! It's also great for controlling our weight. When we eat fiber, it swells up in our stomachs and makes us feel full, which means we're less likely to overeat. It takes longer to digest, so it keeps us feeling satisfied for longer. That's a big help in preventing us from packing on extra pounds and becoming overweight or obese.

Fiber even has an impact on our blood sugar levels. Foods high in fiber take longer to break down, which means they release their sugar into our blood more slowly. That helps keep our blood sugar levels stable, which is important for preventing diabetes. People with diabetes can especially benefit from a fiber-rich diet because it helps keep their blood sugar from spiking and dropping.

And here's another cool thing about fiber: It can help lower cholesterol and keep our hearts healthy. Fiber binds to cholesterol in our guts and helps get rid of it. Some types of fiber, like pectin, oat beta-glucan, and guar gum, are particularly good at lowering LDL cholesterol (the "bad" kind). By reducing our LDL cholesterol levels, fiber lowers our risk of heart attacks, strokes, and other heart problems.

But it's not just about the health benefits—fiber adds variety and goodness to our diet. We can find fiber in lots of different foods, like whole grains, beans, fruits, veggies, nuts, and seeds. By eating these fiber-rich foods, we get a good mix of nutrients and keep our diet balanced. The general recommendation is to aim for 25 to 38 grams of fiber each day, depending on our age and gender.

If we want to increase our fiber intake, here are some tips: Start slowly by adding fiber-rich foods little by little. Choose whole grains instead of refined grains and go for fruits and veggies with the skin on since that's where a lot of the fiber is. Beans, lentils, and chickpeas are also fantastic sources of fiber, so we can toss them into soups, salads, or have them as a side dish. And don't forget about nuts and seeds— they're not only packed with fiber but also healthy fats and proteins. Sprinkle them on salads or yogurt, or enjoy them as a snack.

Oh, and it's important to stay hydrated when we increase our fiber intake. Fiber absorbs water to do its thing, so we need to make sure we're drinking enough water to keep our digestion running smoothly.

All in all, fiber is a big deal for our health and should be a key part of our diet. It keeps our gut healthy, helps us maintain a healthy weight, keeps our blood sugar in check, and reduces the risk of heart problems. By eating fiber-rich foods, we can keep our diet diverse and promote long-term good health.

Getting to know fiber-rich foods:

Fiber is an important component of a healthy diet and plays a crucial role in maintaining optimal digestion and overall good health. It's a type of carbohydrate found in plant-based foods that can't be fully digested by the body. Instead, they mostly pass through the digestive tract unchanged, offering numerous benefits to our bodies.

To reap the health benefits of fiber, it's important to incorporate fiber-rich foods into our diet. Here are some examples of fiber-rich foods that can help increase your daily fiber intake:

1. Whole grains:
Whole grain products like oats, whole wheat bread, brown rice, whole grain pasta, and quinoa are excellent sources of fiber. They contain the entire grain, including the fiber-rich bran and germ. When shopping for grain products, look for the "whole grain" label to ensure you're choosing the fiber-rich option.

2. Legumes:

Beans, lentils, chickpeas, and peas are rich in fiber and also provide a good source of protein. They can be used in soups, stews, salads, or as the main component of vegetarian dishes. Experiment with different varieties to discover a range of flavors and textures.

3. Fruit:
Fruit is not only delicious but also rich in fiber. Apples, pears, berries, oranges, and kiwis are just some examples of fiber-rich fruits. Enjoy them as a healthy snack, add them to cereal or yogurt, or use them in smoothies.

4. Vegetables:
Vegetables are an excellent source of fiber. Broccoli, carrots, spinach, celery, bell peppers, and artichokes are just a few examples of fiber-rich vegetables. Add them to salads, soups, stir-fries, or grilled vegetables to boost your fiber intake.

5. Nuts and seeds:
Nuts and seeds are not only rich in healthy fats and proteins but also in fiber. Almonds, walnuts, chia seeds, flaxseeds, and hemp seeds are good options. Add them as toppings to yogurt, cereal, or salads, or enjoy them as a snack.

6. Oats:
Oats are not only a popular breakfast choice but also an excellent source of fiber. They contain both soluble and insoluble fiber, which contribute to regulating blood sugar levels and providing long-lasting satiety. Enjoy oats as warm porridge, overnight oats, or add them to baked goods like muffins or cookies.

7. Chia and flaxseeds:
Chia and flaxseeds are small but mighty fiber-rich seeds. They can be used in yogurt, smoothies, cereal, or baked goods. They are also a good source of omega-3 fatty acids, which have anti-inflammatory properties.

By incorporating fiber-rich foods into your diet, you can not only increase your fiber intake but also reap the numerous health benefits. Fiber contributes to promoting healthy digestion, controlling blood sugar levels, managing weight, and reducing the risk of heart disease and colon cancer. It's recommended to consume between 25 and 38 grams of fiber daily, depending on age, gender, and individual needs.

A balanced diet that is rich in fiber-rich foods can help you feel fuller for longer, stabilize energy levels, and improve digestive health. Experiment with different fiber-rich foods and recipes to cater to your taste preferences while ensuring optimal fiber intake.

The chapter "The Importance of Fiber" shows us how crucial fiber is for a healthy diet. Fiber-rich foods such as whole grains, legumes, fruit, vegetables, nuts, seeds, oats, and chia and flaxseeds offer numerous health benefits. By integrating these foods into our diet, we can increase our fiber intake and support optimal digestion, blood sugar stability, satiety, and weight control. Fiber also contributes to reducing the risk of heart disease and colon cancer. By enjoying fiber-rich foods and trying out diverse recipes, we can fully harness the benefits of a fiber-rich diet and contribute to our overall health.

Chapter 9: Sugar and Sweet Alternatives

The Effects of Sugar on Health:

Sugar is everywhere in our modern diet, and many people consume it in large quantities, often without realizing it. While sugar offers a sweet temptation, it's important to be aware of the effects of excessive sugar consumption on health.

High consumption of added sugar is associated with a range of health problems. One of the most obvious effects is weight gain. Sugar-laden foods provide many empty calories that offer little to no nutrients but can contribute to a calorie surplus. This can lead to long-term weight gain and an increased risk of obesity. Additionally, excessive sugar consumption can lead to insulin resistance and type 2 diabetes as the body struggles to effectively regulate blood sugar levels.

Sugar can also have negative effects on dental health. Bacteria in the oral cavity feed on sugar and produce acids that attack tooth enamel, leading to cavities. Regular consumption of sugar-sweetened beverages like soda and sweetened tea can significantly increase the risk of cavities.

Furthermore, high sugar intake can contribute to increased inflammation in the body. Chronic inflammation is associated with various health problems, including cardiovascular disease, diabetes, cancer, and autoimmune diseases.

It's important to understand that not all sources of sugar are equal. Natural sugars found in fruits and dairy products usually come with other nutrients like fiber, vitamins, and minerals that support a healthy diet. It's the added sugars found in many processed foods, candies, cakes, pastries, soft drinks, and sweetened beverages that should be avoided.

To reduce sugar consumption, you can turn to natural alternatives that offer sweetness with fewer health impacts. Here are some sweet alternatives to refined sugar:

1. Fruit:
Fresh or dried fruit can provide natural sweetness while also containing fiber and other important nutrients. Berries, apples, bananas, dates, and raisins are good options.

2. Honey:
Honey is a natural sweetener with antioxidant and anti-inflammatory properties. However, it should still be used in moderation as it still contains sugar.

3. Maple syrup:
Maple syrup is derived from the sap of maple trees and contains a variety of minerals such as potassium, calcium, and manganese.

4. Stevia:
Stevia is a plant-based sweetener extracted from the leaves of the Stevia plant. It is calorie-free and does not impact blood sugar levels.

It's important to read food labels and watch out for hidden sugars in processed products. Sugar can appear under different names such as sucrose, fructose, high-fructose corn syrup, or dextrose. By consciously controlling your sugar intake and choosing natural alternatives, you can minimize the negative effects of excessive sugar on health and contribute to a balanced diet.

Tips for Reducing Sugar Consumption:

Excessive sugar consumption can have negative effects on health, increasing the risk of conditions like obesity, type 2 diabetes, heart disease, and cavities. Therefore, it's important to reduce sugar intake and choose healthier alternatives. Here are some detailed tips on how to control your sugar consumption:

1. Raise awareness:
Start by becoming aware of how much sugar you consume daily. Read food labels carefully to identify the sugar content in processed foods. Remember that sugar can appear under various names such as sucrose, fructose, high-fructose corn syrup, or dextrose. By educating yourself about hidden sugars, you can better control how much sugar you actually consume.

2. Choose natural alternatives:

Instead of reaching for sugary snacks, candies, and desserts, opt for natural alternatives that provide a sweet taste. Fresh fruits like berries, apples, bananas, or oranges are delicious and healthy options. They contain natural sugars along with fiber, vitamins, and minerals that are important for the body. Dried fruits like dates, raisins, or figs are also natural sweeteners that can add a sweet touch. They also provide fiber and other nutrients.

3. Cook at home:

By preparing your meals at home, you have control over the ingredients and can reduce the sugar content. Avoid sugar-laden sauces, dressings, and ready-made meals as they often contain hidden sugars. Instead, you can prepare homemade dressings and sauces using healthy ingredients like olive oil, lemon juice, herbs, and spices. This way, you can control the taste and reduce the need for additional sugar.

4. Choose beverages wisely:

Soft drinks, sweetened juices, and energy drinks are often primary sources of added sugar. Opt for water, unsweetened tea, homemade smoothies, or freshly squeezed juice to quench your thirst. If you want to add a sweet touch to your drink, you can squeeze a few drops of lemon or lime juice. You can also rely on herbal teas that naturally have a pleasant sweetness without the need for extra sugar.

5. Gradual reduction:

Instead of abruptly cutting out sugar, you can gradually reduce your sugar intake. Start by reducing or eliminating sugar in your coffee or tea. Also, avoid sugary snacks and candies as between-meal treats. By gradually consuming less sugar, your taste buds will adapt to lower sweetness levels, and over time, you'll have fewer cravings for sugar.

6. Alternative sweeteners:

If you still want sweet flavors in your foods and beverages, you can turn to alternative sweeteners. Natural sweeteners like stevia, erythritol, xylitol, or coconut sugar are healthier options compared to refined sugar. However, keep in mind that these sweeteners should also be used in moderation.

7. Stress management:

People often turn to sugary foods to cope with stress or negative emotions. Look for alternative ways to deal with stress, such as exercise, meditation, relaxation techniques, or pursuing hobbies. By applying healthy coping strategies, you can reduce the emotional connection between stress and sugar consumption.

By following these tips, you can reduce your sugar intake and achieve a healthier diet. It may take some time and adjustment, but the benefits of a balanced diet with reduced sugar are immense. You'll have more energy, better weight control, and long-term improvements in overall health.

Chapter 10: Salt and Its Effects

The Role of Salt in Our Diet:

Salt is one of the basic ingredients in our diet and plays a significant role in enhancing the taste and preserving food. It mainly consists of sodium chloride and provides essential minerals for our body. Salt enhances the flavor of food and contributes to the sensory experience of dishes. It can bring out the flavors and improve the taste of meals. That's because salt stimulates the taste buds on the tongue and intensifies the release of flavors. However, it's important to consume salt in moderation as excessive intake can lead to a dependency on its taste.

Sodium, the main component of salt, is an essential mineral required for various functions in the body. It helps maintain fluid balance, supports kidney function, and plays a role in muscle contraction. However, the body only needs a limited amount of sodium, and excessive consumption can cause health problems.

Excessive salt intake can raise blood pressure, especially in sensitive individuals. Sodium binds water in the body, increasing blood volume, which leads to increased pressure in the blood vessels. Over time, high blood pressure can increase the risk of cardiovascular diseases, strokes, and kidney problems. A salt-rich diet can also impose a higher burden on the kidneys as they have to filter more water to eliminate excess sodium.

High salt consumption can also result in increased calcium excretion through the kidneys. This can contribute to a higher long-term risk of developing osteoporosis, a condition that leads to reduced bone density and an increased risk of fractures. Additionally, a salt-rich diet can raise the risk of kidney stones since excess sodium promotes the formation of crystals in the kidneys.

A salt-rich diet can also cause fluid retention as sodium binds water in the body. This can lead to swelling in the extremities and increase the risk of hypertension and heart failure.

To reduce salt intake and maintain a healthy diet, the following tips can be helpful: Read the nutritional information on food labels to check the salt content of products. Choose fresh foods instead of processed ones, as they often have higher salt content. Use herbs and spices to enhance the flavor of dishes instead of relying on salty seasonings. Rinse preserved foods like pickled vegetables to remove excess salt. Prepare your meals at home to have control over the ingredients and reduce salt content.

It's important to note that salt also exists in many hidden sources, such as snacks, ready-to-eat meals, sauces, and dressings. Therefore, carefully read the ingredient list and opt for low-salt or salt-free alternatives. Also, pay attention to your personal taste preferences and gradually adjust to a reduced salt intake to adapt your taste.

By controlling salt consumption and maintaining a balanced diet, you can help reduce the risk of health problems associated with excessive salt intake and promote a healthy lifestyle.

Tips for Moderate Salt Consumption:

Salt is an essential part of our diet, but excessive consumption can lead to health problems. Therefore, it's important to keep salt intake in moderation and make a conscious decision about how much salt we consume daily.

Excessive salt consumption can contribute to high blood pressure, which is a risk factor for heart disease, strokes, and kidney issues. To reduce salt intake and maintain a healthy diet, the following tips can be helpful:

1. Read the nutrition labels on food:
Check the salt content of products before purchasing them. Choose foods with low salt content or look for low-salt alternatives.

2. Use fresh ingredients:
Fresh foods like fruits, vegetables, lean meat, and fish naturally contain less salt than processed foods. Try to prepare your meals with fresh ingredients to reduce salt content.

3. Season with herbs and spices:
Instead of salt, flavor your dishes with various herbs and spices. Experiment with garlic, onions, lemon juice, lemon zest, paprika, turmeric, and other spices to enhance the taste.

4. Rinse preserved foods:

Preserved foods like pickled vegetables or canned beans can have high salt content. By thoroughly rinsing them, you can remove some of the excess salt.

5. Avoid salt-laden condiments:
Some condiments, such as soy sauce or pre-made seasoning mixes, contain high amounts of salt. Try switching to low-salt alternatives or reduce the use of these condiments.

6. Cook at home:
When you prepare your meals at home, you have full control over the ingredients and salt content. Try different recipes and adjust the amount of salt according to your personal taste.

7. Watch out for hidden salt:
Salt is hidden in many processed foods, such as ready-to-eat meals, snacks, soups, and sauces. Carefully read the ingredient list and choose low-salt or salt-free alternatives.

8. Gradually adapt to reduced salt intake:
Gradually reduce the salt content in your meals to get accustomed to the taste. Your taste buds will adjust over time, and you'll come to appreciate the natural flavors of the food more.

By following these tips and being mindful of your salt consumption, you can help reduce the risk of health problems and promote a healthy diet. A balanced diet with moderate salt intake is an important step towards a healthy lifestyle.

Chapter 11: The Importance of Drinking Enough Water

Why Drinking Enough is Important:

Water is crucial for our body and plays a vital role in many essential functions. Our body consists mostly of water, and it's important to drink enough of it to keep our body healthy and functioning properly.

One of the main goals of drinking enough water is to keep our body adequately hydrated. Water helps to keep the body hydrated, which is essential for the smooth functioning of our organs and systems. It facilitates the transport of nutrients to cells, regulates body temperature, eliminates waste products, and lubricates joints and tissues.

Drinking enough water also supports digestion and metabolism. Water helps in diluting digestive juices, facilitating the breakdown of food and absorption of nutrients. It can also aid in preventing constipation by softening the stool and keeping the digestive tract functioning smoothly. Additionally, adequate water intake can boost metabolism, thus aiding in weight control.

Furthermore, water plays a crucial role in skin health. Sufficient fluid intake can help moisturize the skin, keeping it supple and reducing dryness and wrinkles. It can also help minimize skin issues such as acne and irritation by flushing out toxins from the body and promoting healthy circulation.

Drinking enough water is also important for cognitive function and maintaining optimal mental performance. Studies have shown that mild dehydration can lead to concentration problems, memory impairment, and reduced mental clarity. On the other hand, adequate fluid intake can support brain function and help us stay focused, alert, and perform better mentally.

There isn't an exact amount of water that every person should drink daily as it depends on various factors like body weight, physical activity, climate, and individual needs. However, a general guideline is to drink about 8 glasses (approximately 2 liters) of water daily. During intense physical activity or in hot environments, the fluid requirement may be higher.

It's important to note that water is the best choice to meet your fluid needs. Other beverages like tea, coffee, fruit juices, and sodas can also provide fluids, but they may also contain additional sugar and calories. It's advisable to limit the consumption of sugary drinks and focus on water as the primary source of hydration.

Overall, drinking enough water is of great importance for maintaining a healthy body and optimal health. It supports hydration, digestion, metabolism, skin health, and mental performance. Make sure to meet your fluid needs by regularly drinking water and paying attention to your body's needs.

Tips to Increase Water Intake:

Getting enough fluids, especially water, is super important for our health and well-being. Our body is mostly made up of water, and it plays a crucial role in many bodily functions. It helps regulate body temperature, flush out toxins, support metabolism, and keep our organs functioning properly.

Despite the importance of water, many people struggle to drink enough of it. Here are some tips to boost your water intake:

1. Carry a water bottle with you:
A simple way to remind yourself to drink water regularly is by carrying a water bottle with you. Choose a bottle you like and enjoy having it with you. This way, you'll always have water readily available and can drink it anytime.

2. Set hydration goals:
Set daily hydration goals and strive to achieve them. For example, you can decide to drink a large glass of water before breakfast, have a glass of water before each meal, or take a sip of water every few hours. Setting goals can help you become more mindful of your water consumption.

3. Use flavor enhancers:
Some people find plain water boring or unappealing. If that's the case, you can add some flavor to your water to make it more enticing. Try adding fresh lemon or cucumber slices, mint leaves, or berries. This gives the water a refreshing taste without adding extra sugar or calories.

4. Drink water before meals:
Have a glass of water before every meal. This has several benefits. Firstly, it helps increase your water intake. Secondly, it can make you feel fuller faster, leading to eating less and potentially aiding in weight loss.

5. Set reminders:
In our busy lives, we sometimes forget to drink enough water. Set reminders on your smartphone or schedule alarms to remind you to drink water regularly. You can also place small notes in places where you frequently see them, such as on the fridge or your desk.

6. Drink water on every occasion:
Take every opportunity to drink water. When you leave the house, bring a water bottle with you. If you work in an office, always keep a glass of water on your desk. By making water a habit and drinking it regularly, it becomes a natural part of your routine.

7. Experiment with temperatures:
Some people prefer cold water, while others enjoy warm or even hot water. Find out which temperature is most pleasant for you and drink your water in that form. You can also experiment with different temperatures and see what works best for you.

8. Eat water-rich foods:

In addition to drinking water, you can increase your water intake by incorporating water-rich foods into your diet. Fruits like watermelon, grapes, and oranges, as well as vegetables like cucumbers, tomatoes, and bell peppers, have high water content. Consuming these foods regularly contributes to your fluid intake.

9. Make water drinking a habit:
Habits form when we do something regularly. Make it a goal to make drinking enough water a habit. Always have a water bottle with you, drink a glass of water before meals, and regularly remind yourself to drink enough. Over time, it will become easier for you to consume enough water.

By following these tips and being mindful of your water intake, you can increase your fluid consumption and benefit from the many health advantages that come with drinking enough water. Remember that everyone's body is different and has individual needs. Listen to your body and adjust your water intake accordingly.

Chapter 12: Putting Together a Balanced Meal

Building a Balanced Meal:

Putting together a balanced meal is a fundamental step toward a healthy diet. It's about combining the right nutrients in the right amounts to provide the body with the energy and building blocks it needs to function optimally. The basics of a balanced meal include carbohydrates, proteins, healthy fats, fiber, vitamins, and minerals.

Carbohydrates are an important source of energy for the body. They provide glucose, which is the main fuel for our cells. Whole grain products like whole wheat bread, oats, whole wheat pasta, and brown rice are good sources of complex carbohydrates. These are digested more slowly and help stabilize blood sugar levels. Fruits and vegetables also contain carbohydrates but in the form of simple sugars combined with fiber, vitamins, and minerals.

Proteins are the body's building blocks and are essential for tissue growth and repair. They can be found in meat, fish, poultry, eggs, dairy products, legumes such as beans and lentils, as well as nuts and seeds. It's important to combine different protein sources to get all the essential amino acids that the body needs.

Healthy fats play an important role in the diet. They are rich in energy and contribute to the absorption of fat-soluble vitamins. Unsaturated fats, found in avocados, nuts, seeds, and plant oils like olive oil and canola oil, are particularly beneficial for heart and vascular health. Saturated fats, mainly found in animal products like meat and dairy, should be consumed in moderation. Trans fats, found in many processed foods, should be avoided.

Fiber is an essential component of a balanced meal. It contributes to digestive health, helps regulate blood sugar levels, and provides a long-lasting feeling of fullness. Fiber-rich foods include whole grain products, legumes, fruits, vegetables, nuts, and seeds. By incorporating these into meals, you increase nutrient density and support healthy digestion.

Vitamins and minerals are essential for many functions in the body. Fruits and vegetables are rich in vitamins and minerals, providing a variety of nutrients, including vitamin C, vitamin A, potassium, and magnesium. Dairy products supply calcium, while whole grain products and legumes are a good source of B vitamins and iron. Choosing a diverse range of foods in different colors ensures a balanced intake of vitamins and minerals.

To create a balanced meal, individual needs and preferences should be taken into account. It's important to be mindful of any food intolerances or allergies. Meals should not only be balanced but also tasty and appealing. It's advisable to reduce the consumption of added sugar, saturated fats, and heavily processed foods.

By considering the basics of a balanced meal and choosing a variety of foods from different categories, you can ensure that your body receives all the necessary nutrients. A balanced diet is a crucial part of a healthy lifestyle in the long run and supports overall well-being and health.

Tips for Portion Control:

Putting together a balanced meal is a step toward healthy eating. It's about combining the right nutrients in the right amount to provide the body with the energy and building blocks it needs. In addition to choosing the right foods, portion control is also important. Here are some tips to keep portion sizes in check:

1. Use smaller plates:
Swap out large plates for smaller ones. This makes the portions appear larger, giving you the feeling of eating more even though you're actually consuming less.

2. Mind the recommended portions:

Refer to the recommended portions for different food groups. A rule of thumb, for example, is that a serving of meat or fish should be the size of your palm.

3. Use measuring cups and scales:
Use measuring cups and kitchen scales to measure the exact amount of food. This gives you a better sense of portion sizes and helps you avoid overeating.

4. Share meals:
When dining out or preparing a large meal at home, share it with another person. This helps reduce portions and prevents overeating.

5. Pay attention to your satiety signals:
Eat slowly and pay attention to your body's signals telling you when you're full. Stop eating when you feel satisfied and not excessively full.

6. Fill your plate with vegetables:
Vegetables are low in calories and high in fiber. So, fill a large portion of your plate with vegetables to increase the overall volume of the meal without consuming excessive calories.

7. Limit the use of sauces and dressings:
Sauces and dressings can quickly add calories. Use them sparingly and opt for low-fat or homemade versions whenever possible.

8. Plan your meals in advance:
By planning your meals in advance, you can better control portion sizes and avoid unhealthy choices.

9. Mind the snack portions:
It's important to keep portion sizes in mind even when snacking. Pack snacks in portioned sizes to prevent overeating.

10. Pay attention to your hunger and satiety signals:
Take time to eat mindfully and pay attention to your hunger and satiety signals. Eat when you're hungry and stop eating when you're full.

Portion control is an important aspect of a balanced meal. By consciously paying attention to portion sizes and following these tips, you can better control your diet and promote a healthy lifestyle.

Chapter 13: Healthy Snacks for In-Between

<u>Nutritious Snack Options</u>:

Healthy snacks for in-between are a great way to satisfy hunger, boost energy, and rev up metabolism without resorting to unhealthy options. Here are some nutritious snack options you can incorporate into your diet:

<u>1. Fresh fruit</u>:
Fruit is an excellent choice for a healthy snack. It's rich in vitamins, minerals, fiber, and antioxidants. Choose seasonal fruits like apples, bananas, berries, oranges, or grapes and enjoy them as a snack.

<u>2. Veggie sticks with dip</u>:
Crisp vegetables like carrots, bell peppers, cucumbers, or celery are great for snacking. Pair them with healthy dips like hummus, guacamole, or Greek yogurt for added flavor and nutrients.

<u>3. Nuts and seeds</u>:
Nuts and seeds are packed with healthy fats, proteins, and fiber. Almonds, walnuts, chia seeds, flaxseeds, or sunflower seeds are good options for an energy-boosting snack. However, watch out for portion sizes as they are calorie-dense.

<u>4. Greek yogurt</u>:
Greek yogurt is a protein-rich and creamy snack option. It also provides calcium and probiotic cultures that can promote digestion. Add fresh fruit, nuts, or a drizzle of honey to vary the taste.

<u>5. Whole grain crackers with hummus</u>:
Whole grain crackers are high in fiber and provide a good base for a snack. Pair them with hummus, a healthy source of plant-based protein, fiber, and healthy fats.

<u>6. Hard-boiled eggs</u>:
Hard-boiled eggs are a protein-rich option for a snack. They also contain important nutrients like vitamin D and choline. You can eat them on their own or slice them and place them on whole grain bread.

<u>7. Cottage cheese with fruits</u>:
Cottage cheese is a protein-rich alternative to yogurt and contains less sugar. Combine it with fresh fruits like berries, pineapple, or peaches for a healthy and satisfying snack.

<u>8. Oatmeal bars</u>:

Homemade oatmeal bars are a healthy snack option that you can customize to your liking. Use oats, nuts, dried fruits, and healthy sweeteners like honey or maple syrup to create nutritious bars.

9. Vegetable soup:
A warm vegetable soup can be a filling and nutritious option for a snack. Prepare a homemade vegetable soup using fresh vegetables and healthy broths.

10. Dark chocolate:
Dark chocolate with a high cocoa content is rich in antioxidants and can be a healthy alternative to sweet snacks. Enjoy it in moderation and choose varieties with low sugar content.

When choosing healthy snacks, it's important to pay attention to the quality of ingredients and portion sizes. Experiment with different options to cater to your individual taste and preferences. By opting for nutritious snacks, you can promote your health and stay energized throughout the day.

Ideas for healthy snack:

1. Tuna-Stuffed Cucumber Boats:

- Ingredients:
  - 1 large cucumber
  - 1 can of water-packed tuna (drained)
  - 2 tablespoons of Greek yogurt
  - 1 tablespoon of lemon juice
  - 1 tablespoon of chopped fresh herbs (such as parsley, dill)
  - Salt and pepper to taste

- Preparation:
  1. Cut the cucumber in half lengthwise and remove the seeds with a spoon to form a boat-like shape.
  2. In a bowl, mix the drained tuna, Greek yogurt, lemon juice, and chopped herbs.
  3. Season with salt and pepper.
  4. Fill the cucumber halves with the tuna mixture.
  5. Slice the filled cucumbers and serve them as a refreshing and protein-rich snack.

2. Quinoa Energy Balls:

- Ingredients:
  - 1 cup of cooked quinoa
  - 1/2 cup of oats
  - 1/4 cup of honey or maple syrup
  - 1/4 cup of almond butter
  - 1/4 cup of chopped nuts (such as almonds, walnuts)
  - 1/4 cup of dried fruits (such as raisins, cranberries)
  - 1 teaspoon of vanilla extract
  - 1 teaspoon of cinnamon

- Preparation:
  1. In a bowl, thoroughly mix all the ingredients until well combined.
  2. Place the mixture in the refrigerator for about 30 minutes to firm up.
  3. Shape the mixture into small balls.
  4. Store the energy balls in the refrigerator and enjoy them as a healthy snack whenever needed.

3. Caprese Skewers
:

- Ingredients:
  - Cherry tomatoes
  - Mozzarella balls
  - Fresh basil leaves
  - Olive oil
  - Balsamic glaze
  - Salt and pepper to taste

- Preparation:
  1. Thread a cherry tomato, a mozzarella ball, and a basil leaf onto wooden skewers.
  2. Arrange the skewers on a serving plate.
  3. Drizzle olive oil and balsamic glaze over the skewers.
  4. Season with salt and pepper.
  5. Enjoy these refreshing and flavorful Caprese skewers as a healthy snack.

4. Banana Oat Cookies:

- Ingredients:

- 2 ripe bananas
- 1 1/2 cups of oats
- 1/4 cup of raisins or chopped dried fruits
- 1/4 cup of chopped nuts (such as almonds, walnuts)
- 1 teaspoon of cinnamon
- 1 teaspoon of vanilla extract

- Preparation:
  1. Preheat the oven to 180°C and line a baking sheet with parchment paper.
  2. In a bowl, mash the bananas.
  3. Add oats, raisins, chopped nuts, cinnamon, and vanilla extract. Mix well.
  4. Drop spoonfuls of the dough onto the baking sheet and flatten slightly.
  5. Bake the cookies for about 15-20 minutes until golden brown.
  6. Allow them to cool and enjoy these healthy and delicious banana oat cookies.

5. Greek Yogurt with Nuts and Honey:

- Ingredients:
  - Greek yogurt
  - Chopped nuts (such as almonds, walnuts, cashews)
  - Honey

- Preparation:
  1. Take a bowl and fill it with Greek yogurt.
  2. Sprinkle chopped nuts over the yogurt.
  3. Drizzle some honey over the nuts.
  4. Mix everything well and enjoy this creamy and nutritious snack.

6. Vegetable Sticks with Hummus:

- Ingredients:
  - Assorted vegetables (such as carrots, celery, bell peppers, cucumbers)
  - Hummus

- Preparation:
  1. Cut the vegetables into sticks or slices.
  2. Serve the vegetables with a bowl of hummus as a dip.
  3. Dip the vegetable sticks in the hummus and enjoy this crunchy and protein-rich snack option.

7. Oatmeal Banana Muffins:
  - Ingredients:

- 2 ripe bananas
- 1 cup of oats
- 1/2 cup of almond milk or other plant-based milk
- 1 tablespoon of honey or maple syrup
- 1 teaspoon of baking powder
- 1 teaspoon of cinnamon

- Preparation:
  1. Preheat the oven to 180°C and place muffin liners on a baking sheet.
  2. In a bowl, mash the bananas.
  3. Add oats, almond milk, honey, baking powder, and cinnamon. Mix well.
  4. Fill the muffin liners with the batter and bake for about 20-25 minutes until golden brown.
  5. Let the muffins cool and enjoy them as a tasty and satisfying snack.

8. Edamame Salad:

- Ingredients:
  - Edamame (soybeans) - frozen or fresh
  - Cherry tomatoes (halved)
  - Cucumbers (diced)
  - Spring onions (thinly sliced)
  - Lemon juice
  - Olive oil
  - Salt and pepper to taste

- Preparation:
  1. Cook the edamame according to the package instructions and let them cool.
  2. In a bowl, combine the edamame, cherry tomatoes, cucumbers, and spring onions.
  3. Season with lemon juice, olive oil, salt, and pepper.
  4. Mix well and serve the edamame salad as a refreshing and protein-rich snack.

9. Avocado Egg Salad:

- Ingredients:
  - 1 ripe avocado (pitted and mashed)
  - 2 hard-boiled eggs (chopped)
  - 1 tablespoon of Greek yogurt
  - 1 tablespoon of lemon juice
  - 1 tablespoon of chopped fresh herbs (such as parsley, chives)
  - Salt and pepper to taste

- Preparation:
    1. In a bowl, mix the mashed avocado, chopped eggs, Greek yogurt, lemon juice, and chopped herbs.
    2. Season with salt and pepper.
    3. Serve the avocado egg salad on whole grain bread or as a dip for vegetable sticks.

10. Quinoa Chocolate Energy Balls:

- Ingredients:
    - 1 cup of cooked quinoa
    - 1/2 cup of oats
    - 1/4 cup of peanut butter
    - 1/4 cup of honey or maple syrup
    - 1/4 cup of unsweetened cocoa powder
    - 1 teaspoon of vanilla extract
    - Pinch of salt
    - Optional: chopped nuts, raisins, or other dried fruits

- Preparation:
    1. In a bowl, thoroughly mix all the ingredients.
    2. Shape the dough into small balls.
    3. Let the quinoa chocolate energy balls firm up in the refrigerator for about 30 minutes.
    4. Enjoy these delicious and energy-packed snacks that you can take with you.

Try out these recipes and treat yourself to healthy snacks throughout the day!

Chapter 14: Eating Healthy in Everyday Life

Incorporating Healthy Eating into Your Daily Routine:

Eating healthy plays a crucial role in our well-being and health. However, it often seems challenging to integrate a balanced diet into everyday life, especially with a busy lifestyle. Nevertheless, there are various strategies and tips to make healthy eating a habit. Planning is key to a healthy diet in daily life. Take the time to plan meals and snacks in advance. Create a shopping list and purchase fresh, healthy ingredients. Prepare meals and portion them for the coming days. This way, you always have healthy options on hand and avoid impulsive eating.

Preparing meals at home allows you to have control over the ingredients and portion sizes. Experiment with new recipes and discover healthy alternatives to your favorite dishes. Use fresh ingredients, whole grains, lean protein, and healthy fats to prepare balanced meals. Remember that it's not about giving up specific foods but finding a healthy balance.

Snacks are an essential part of a healthy diet. Prepare healthy snacks in advance to avoid cravings. Cut fruits and vegetables into convenient pieces and store them in resealable containers. Nuts, yogurt, whole grain crackers, or homemade energy bars are also good snack options. Pay attention to proper portion sizes and avoid excessive snacking.

Adequate hydration is essential for a healthy diet. Drink water regularly throughout the day. Take a water bottle with you when leaving the house to ensure you drink enough. Alternatively, you can enjoy unsweetened tea or fruit-infused water. Hydration is important to properly support the body and maintain metabolism.

A healthy diet doesn't mean changing everything at once. Start with small steps. For example, replace refined sugar with natural sweeteners like honey or maple syrup. Reduce the consumption of processed foods and instead add more fresh produce to your meals. Slow and steady changes lead to long-term success. Give yourself time to develop new habits and reward yourself for your progress.

Take time for your meals and practice mindful eating. Savor each bite consciously and notice the flavors and textures. Eat slowly and stop when you're full. This helps you develop a better understanding of your body's needs and avoid overeating.

Shared meals are a wonderful opportunity to promote healthy eating habits. Whenever possible, eat together with your family or friends. Shared meals create a positive atmosphere and allow for the exchange of healthy eating habits. Take the time to talk and enjoy the food together.

Integrating a healthy diet into daily life requires time and commitment, but the long-term benefits are worth it. By consciously shaping your diet, you can improve your health and feel energized. Start today and make healthy eating a regular part of your everyday life.

Strategies for Healthy Meals Under Time Pressure:

Eating healthy in a hectic daily life can be a big challenge, especially when time is scarce. However, it is possible to prepare healthy meals and maintain a balanced diet even under time pressure. Here are some practical strategies that can help:

1. Meal Prep:

Set aside regular time to prepare meals for the upcoming week. This can be done on weekends or a day when you have some free time. Use this time to wash and chop vegetables, prepare salads, and cook side dishes like rice or quinoa in advance. Store these prepared ingredients in airtight containers in the fridge for quick access throughout the week. This saves time in meal preparation and keeps healthy ingredients readily available.

2. Quick and Easy Recipes:

Look for recipes that require minimal preparation time. There are numerous quick and healthy dishes that you can prepare in a short amount of time. For example, you can create a healthy Buddha Bowl by combining sautéed vegetables, proteins like chicken or tofu, and a source of healthy fats like avocado. Alternatively, you can fill a whole-grain wrap with fresh vegetables and a protein source such as tuna or hummus. These dishes are quick to prepare and offer a balanced nutritional composition.

3. Leftover Utilization:

Don't let food go to waste. Use leftover ingredients or meals from the previous day to create new dishes. For example, you can transform leftover roasted vegetables into a delicious frittata or omelette. Or use cooked chicken or meat from the previous day to prepare a healthy salad or filling for wraps or sandwiches. Utilizing leftovers not only saves time but also reduces food waste, making it a sustainable option.

4. Quick Snack Options:

Always have healthy snacks on hand that are ready to eat quickly. There are plenty of nutritious snack options that you can easily carry with you or prepare at home. These include nuts, fresh fruits, Greek yogurt, hard-boiled eggs, healthy granola bars, or vegetable sticks with hummus. These snacks provide essential nutrients and keep you satisfied between meals when you have little time to prepare a full meal.

5. Simplify Preparation:

Choose preparation methods that take less time. This includes steaming vegetables, grilling meat or fish, and using pre-cut or frozen vegetables. These methods require less preparation time and still allow you to prepare healthy meals.

Remember that it's important to prioritize your health and make conscious decisions even when you're under time pressure. A balanced diet can help you feel energized and support your long-term health. By applying the strategies mentioned above and taking some time for meal planning and preparation, you can eat healthily even in your busy daily life.

Chapter 15: Sustainable Eating

The Impact of Our Diet on the Environment:

Our diet has a significant impact on the environment. The way we eat and the foods we consume can have direct effects on climate change, resource utilization, water consumption, and biodiversity. Here's a detailed look at the impact of our diet on the environment:

1. Greenhouse Gas Emissions:
Food production, especially animal products like meat and dairy, contributes significantly to the release of greenhouse gases such as carbon dioxide (CO_2) and methane (CH_4). Industrial livestock farming, the use of fertilizers, and the cultivation of animal feed require large amounts of energy and lead to deforestation to make room for agricultural land. By consuming plant-based foods and reducing the consumption of meat and dairy, we can significantly reduce our greenhouse gas emissions.

2. Water Consumption:
Food production requires large amounts of water. In particular, the cultivation of animal feed, such as soy used for livestock, has high water consumption. Generally, the consumption of plant-based foods requires less water compared to animal products. By consciously consuming water and choosing low-water foods such as legumes, grains, and vegetables, we can reduce our water consumption.

3. Land Use and Deforestation:
Agricultural production requires large areas to grow food or raise livestock. This leads to deforestation of natural habitats, especially in tropical regions. Deforestation contributes to a reduction in biodiversity and affects ecosystems. By consuming locally grown foods and supporting sustainable agricultural practices, we can help reduce deforestation and preserve biodiversity.

4. Food Waste:

Another issue related to our diet is food waste. Large quantities of food are discarded annually, resulting in not only financial losses but also a waste of resources and an additional contribution to climate change. By conscious shopping, proper food storage, and creative use of leftovers, we can help reduce food waste.

5. Sustainable Agricultural Practices:
To minimize the impact of our diet on the environment, it is important to support sustainable agricultural practices. These include organic farming, the use of organic fertilizers, water management, and the protection of biodiversity. Consuming organic food and purchasing products from local sustainable agriculture can contribute to promoting a more sustainable diet.

It is crucial that we become aware of how our diet influences the environment and take appropriate measures to eat more sustainably. By prioritizing plant-based foods, reducing food waste, supporting sustainable agriculture, and conscious shopping, we can reduce our ecological footprint and contribute to a healthier and more sustainable future.

Tips for a More Sustainable Eating Approach:

A sustainable eating approach is more than just a healthy diet. It also involves considering the impact of our diet on the environment and the well-being of other beings. Here are some detailed tips on how you can make your diet more sustainable:

- When it comes to food choices, opt for local and seasonal products. By choosing food from your area, you minimize transportation efforts and support local farmers. Additionally, seasonal foods often have higher nutrient content as they are harvested at the optimal time.

- Another step towards sustainable eating is promoting plant-based foods. Plant-based foods generally have a lower environmental impact compared to animal products. Try replacing some of your animal-based foods with plant-based alternatives like legumes, nuts, seeds, and whole grains. This not only contributes to reducing greenhouse gas emissions but can also have positive effects on your health.

- Organic products are another option for a more sustainable eating approach. They are grown considering specific ecological principles and contribute to reducing the use of pesticides and fertilizers. So, choose organic products whenever possible to reduce environmental impact.

- Reducing food waste is also an important aspect of sustainable eating. Plan your meals in advance to limit unnecessary grocery shopping. Store food properly to extend its shelf life, and get creative with leftovers to prepare new dishes. By minimizing food waste, you contribute to resource conservation and save money.

- Another focus is on avoiding single-use packaging. Buy food in reusable containers or in larger quantities to reduce the consumption of disposable packaging. Also, use reusable bags while shopping to avoid plastic bags.

- To reduce water consumption, be mindful of food preparation and dishwashing. Use only as much water as necessary and, if possible, use rainwater or recycled water for plants and gardens.

- Support local agriculture by shopping directly at farmers' markets or participating in Community Supported Agriculture (CSA). By buying directly from farmers, you promote sustainable agriculture and contribute to strengthening the local community.

- Avoid excessive consumption of processed foods. They often require more resources in production and contribute to the generation of packaging waste. Instead, focus on fresh, unprocessed foods that are rich in nutrients and promote a healthy diet.

- Sustainable eating also begins in your own kitchen. Cook your meals at home instead of relying on ready-made meals or fast food. By preparing your own meals, you have control over the ingredients and cooking methods. This not only helps reduce packaging waste but also allows you to enjoy healthy and balanced meals.

- Educate yourself about sustainable eating and share your knowledge with family and friends. Together, you can have a positive impact on the environment and inspire others to make sustainable choices in their diet.

- Sustainable eating requires conscious decisions and ongoing adjustments to our habits. By following these tips and integrating sustainable eating into our daily lives, we can make a significant contribution to reducing our ecological footprints and create a healthier future for our planet and ourselves.

Dear readers,

We've now embarked on a journey through the world of healthy eating together, and I hope you've gained valuable insights along the way. "Simple Explanation of Healthy Nutrition" is part of a book series that aims to present complex topics in an understandable and accessible manner. Because we believe that knowledge is the foundation for positive change.

In today's society, which is flooded with information, it's often challenging to keep track and make informed decisions. The "simple explanation" book series aims to provide you exactly that - easy access to knowledge and information that can enrich and improve your life.

I warmly invite you to continue exploring the "simple explanation" book series and to apply the knowledge you've gained here to other areas of your life. Because healthy eating is just one puzzle piece to a happy and fulfilling life. By engaging with various aspects, we can develop ourselves holistically and enhance our quality of life.

Lastly, I want to thank you for choosing "Simple Explanation of Healthy Nutrition" I hope this book has helped you understand and practically implement the fundamentals of healthy eating. Remember that every small change matters and that it's never too late to make conscious decisions for your health.

I wish you all the best on your journey toward a healthy and fulfilling lifestyle. May this book inspire you to expand your knowledge, establish new habits, and unleash your full potential.

Warm regards,

Kevin van Olafson